Nurse Pharmacology

A Relaxed Study Guide for the Next Gen NCLEX Exam

Volume 3: Respiratory and Antimicrobial Medications

Get a set of flashcards and copies of
pre-publication books for FREE!
Sign Up Today at:
www.nursereadinessacademy.com

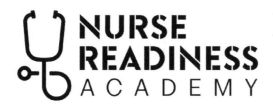 

We value your feedback! Leave a review and show off your artwork!

ISBN: 9798850302085
Copyright © 2023 Nurse Readiness Academy
All Rights Reserved

DISCLAIMER

This coloring book is intended as a reference guide for students, healthcare professionals, and others seeking information on pharmacology. The contents are based on the most current information available at the time of publication, and are intended to provide general information and educational material. This coloring book is not intended to diagnose, treat, cure or prevent any disease or medical condition. If you have any health concerns, you should consult your healthcare professional. The information provided in this coloring book is not intended to replace the advice of a qualified healthcare professional. If you are taking any medications, or have any medical conditions, you should consult your healthcare professional before starting any new treatment. The authors and publishers make no representations or warranties with respect to the accuracy or completeness of the contents of this coloring book and specifically disclaim any implied warranties of merchantability or fitness for a particular purpose. The authors and publishers shall not be held responsible for any errors or omissions, or for any damages resulting from the use of information contained in this coloring book. This coloring book is subject to change without notice, and the authors and publishers do not guarantee that any errors or omissions will be corrected. The information contained is intended for educational purposes only. By using this coloring book, you agree to the terms of this disclaimer. If you do not agree with these terms, you should not use this coloring book.

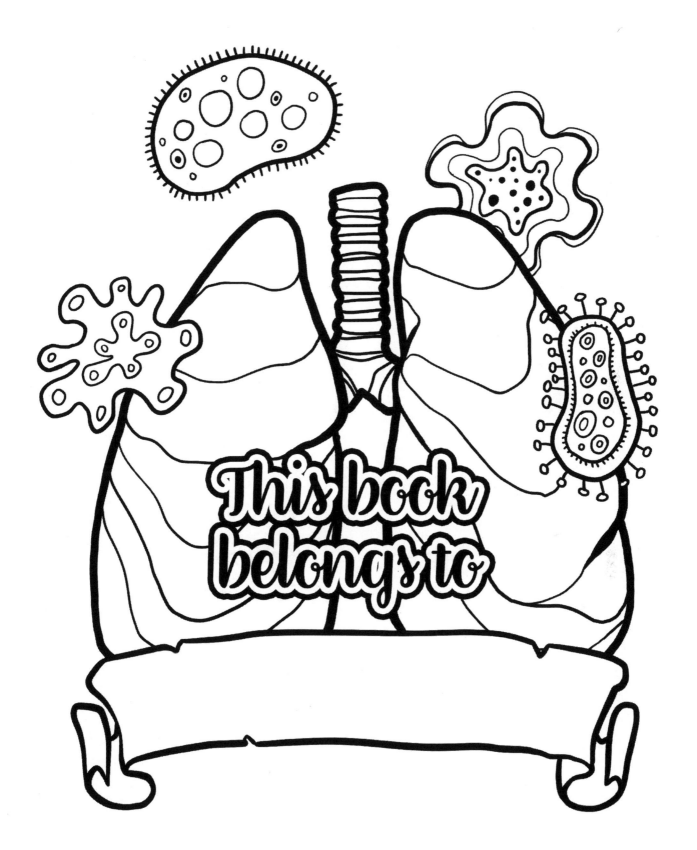

Table of Contents

This book covers the following medications in alphabetical order:

Respiratory

Albuterol
Budesonide
Epoprostenol
Fluticasone
Formoterol
Guaifenesin
Ipratropium
Montelukast
Prednisone
Racemic Epinephrine
Salmeterol
Terbutaline

Antimicrobial

Acyclovir
Amoxicillin
Ampicillin
Azythromycin
Cefaclor
Cefdinir
Cephalexin
Ciprofloxacin
Clindamycin
Erythromycin
Isoniazide
Levofloxacin
Metronidazole
Nystatin
Rifampin
Tetracycline
Trimethoprim/Sulfamethoxazole
Vancomycin

AT A GLANCE

Use the color test page at the back of this book to see what your favorite colors look like on the page. Then, use this page to assign colors to medications grouped by therapeutic class.

Bronchodilator
albuterol
formoterol
ipratropium bromide
racemic epinephrine
salmeterol
terbutaline

Antiasthmatic
fluticasone

Antifungal
nystatin

Antiviral
acyclovir

Anti-inflammatory
budesonide
prednisone

Antibiotic
amoxicillin
ampicillin
azithromycin
cefaclor
cefdinir
cephalexin
clindamycin
erythromycin

Antitubercular
isoniazid
rifampin

Anti-Pulmonary Hypertensive
epoprostenol

Expectorant
guaifenesin

Antibiotic
ciprofloxacin
levofloxacin
tetracycline
trimethoprim / sulfamethoxazole
vancomycin

Antiprotozoal
metronidazole

Therapeutic Class

BRONCHODILATOR

ALBUTEROL

Pharmacologic Class

BETA 2 AGONIST

ALBUTEROL

TRADE NAME
Proventil
Ventolin

INDICATION
Asthma, COPD

ACTION
Beta 2 adrenergic receptor agonist, leading to relaxation of the smooth muscles of the airway

NURSING CONSIDERATIONS
- May decrease effectiveness of beta blockers
- Use caution with heart disease, diabetes, glaucoma, seizures
- Overuse can lead to bronchospasm
- Monitor for chest pain and palpitations
- Can decrease digoxin levels

NOTES

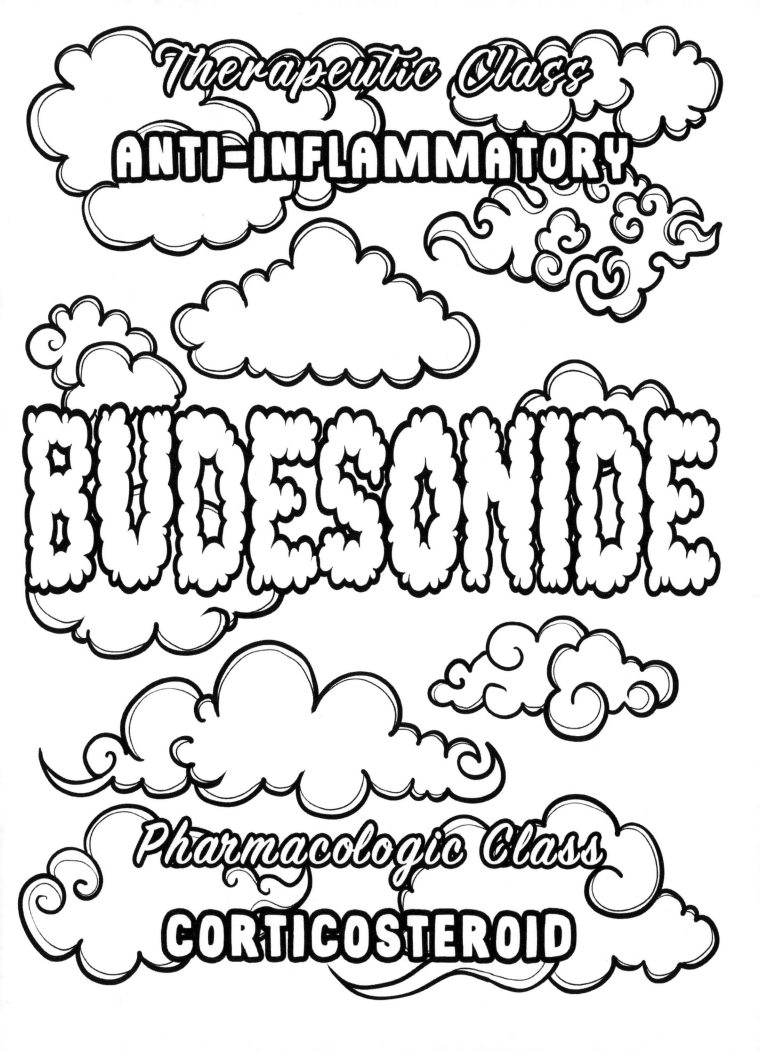

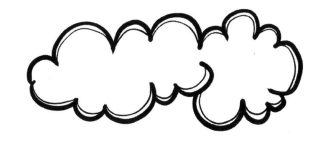

BUDESONIDE

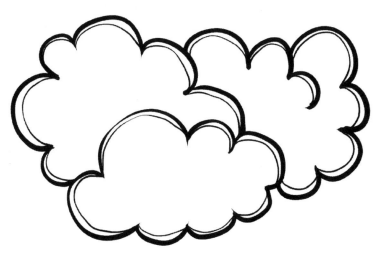

TRADE NAME
Pulmicort

INDICATION
Asthma, COPD

ACTION
Locally acting anti-inflammatory agent

NURSING CONSIDERATIONS
- May cause headache, insomnia, bronchospasm, adrenal suppression
- Use caution with untreated infections and immunosuppressed patients
- Monitor respiratory status
- May lead to decreased bone density
- Instruct patients to use bronchodilators before taking corticosteroids

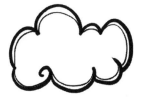

NOTES

_____
_____
_____
_____
_____
_____
_____

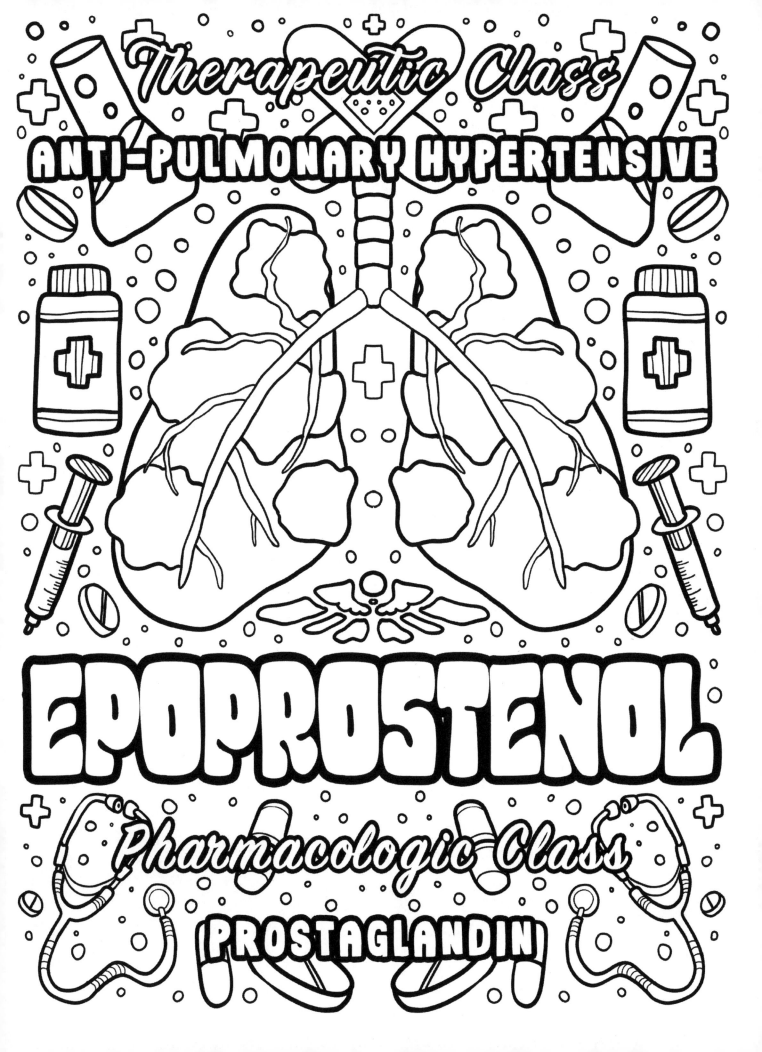

EPOPROSTENOL

TRADE NAME
Flolan

INDICATION
Pulmonary Arterial Hypertension (PAH)

ACTION
Direct vasodilation of pulmonary and systemic arterial vascular beds

NURSING CONSIDERATIONS
- Assess heart rate, ECG, and heart sounds, especially during exercise
- Assess respiratory status
- Monitor for chest pain and palpitations
- DO NOT discontinue abruptly

NOTES

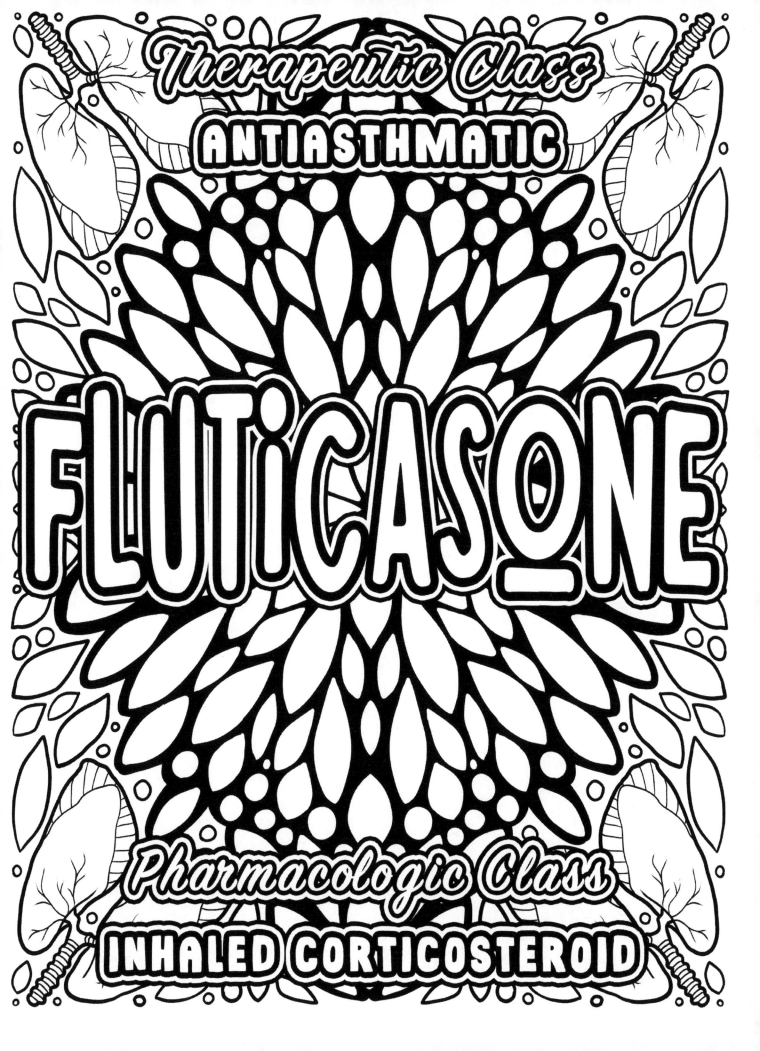

FLUTICASONE

TRADE NAME
Flovent

INDICATION
Asthma prophylaxis

ACTION
Locally acting anti-inflammatory agent

NURSING CONSIDERATIONS
- May cause headache, insomnia, bronchospasm, adrenal suppression
- Use caution with untreated infections and immunosuppressed patients
- Monitor respiratory status
- May lead to decreased bone density
- Instruct patients to use bronchodilators before taking corticosteroids

NOTES

Therapeutic Class
BRONCHODILATOR

FORMOTEROL

Pharmacologic Class
LONG-ACTING BETA AGONIST

FORMOTEROL

TRADE NAME
Foradil

INDICATION
Asthma, COPD

ACTION
Long acting beta 2 adrenergic receptor agonist, leading to relaxation of the smooth muscles of the airway for up to 12 hours

NURSING CONSIDERATIONS
- May decrease effectiveness of beta blockers
- Use caution with heart disease, diabetes, glaucoma, seizures
- Overuse can lead to bronchospasm
- Monitor for chest pain and palpitations
- Can decrease digoxin levels

NOTES

Therapeutic Class

EXPECTORANT

GUAIFENESIN

Pharmacologic Class

MUCOLYTIC

GUAIFENESIN

TRADE NAME
Robitussin

INDICATION
Cough, Congestion

ACTION
Mobilizes secretions and decreases their viscosity

NURSING CONSIDERATIONS
- Instruct patient to avoid taking OTC cold medications
- Assess lung sounds
- Maintain adequate fluid intake

NOTES

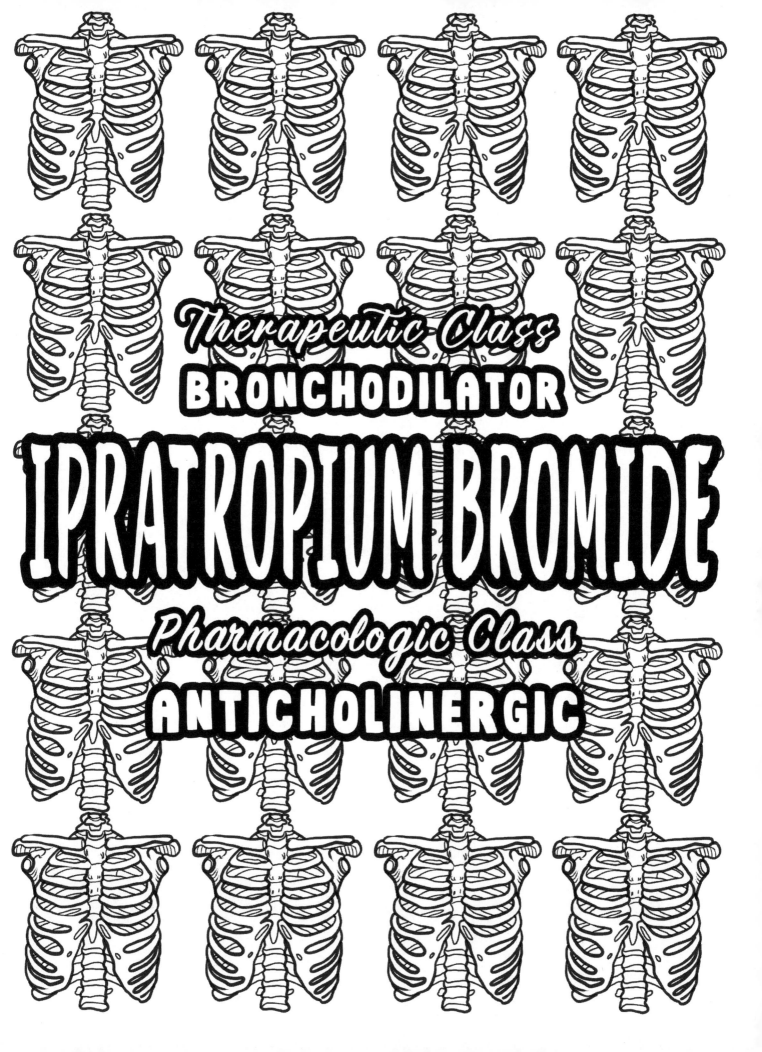

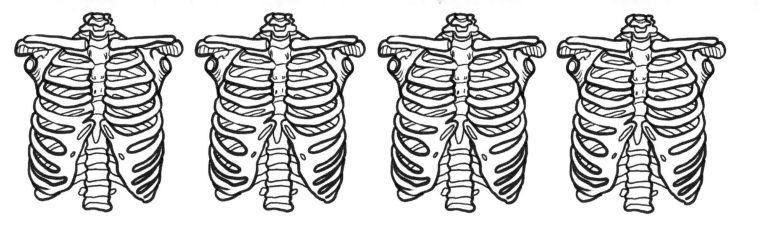

IPRATROPIUM BROMIDE

TRADE NAME
Atrovent

INDICATION
Asthma, COPD, Emphysema

ACTION
Blocks cholinergic receptors, leading to decreased smooth muscle contraction

NOTES

NURSING CONSIDERATIONS

- Use nebulizer mouthpiece instead of face mask to avoid blurred vision or aggravation of narrow-angle glaucoma.
- Ensure adequate hydration, control environmental temperature to prevent hyperpyrexia.
- Have patient void before taking medication to avoid urinary retention.
- Teach patient proper use of inhaler.
- May cause Dizziness, headache, blurred vision, nausea/vomiting, cough, palpitations

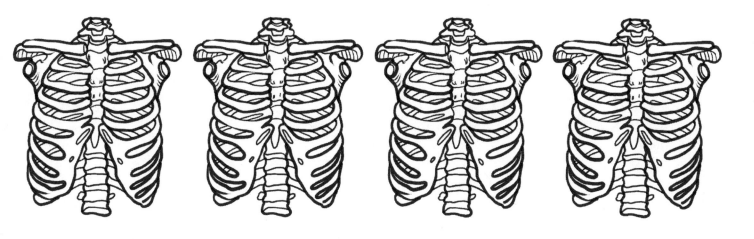

Therapeutic Class
BRONCHODILATOR

MONTELUKAST

Pharmacologic Class
LEUKOTRIENE ANTAGONIST

MONTELUKAST

TRADE NAME
Singulair

INDICATION
Asthma, Seasonal Allergies, Exercise-Induced Bronchoconstriction

ACTION
Disrupts leukotriene activity, decreasing airway edema and smooth muscle constriction

NURSING CONSIDERATIONS
- Assess respiratory status
- Assess liver function
- DO NOT USE for acute asthma attacks

NOTES
_____
_____
_____
_____
_____
_____
_____
_____

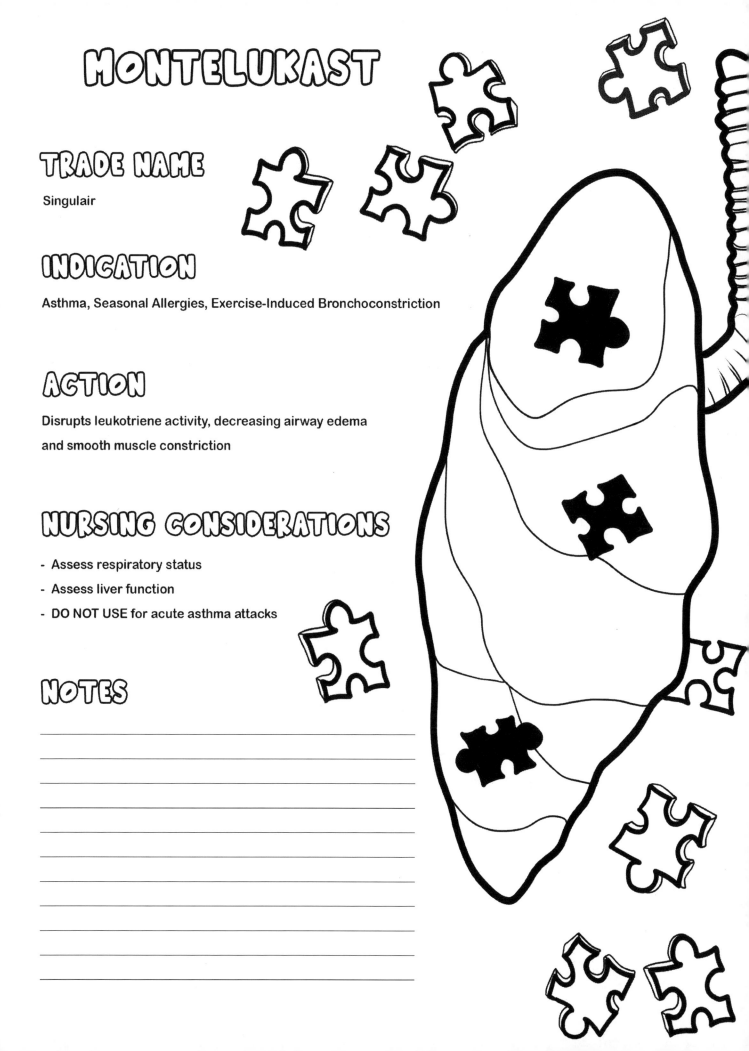

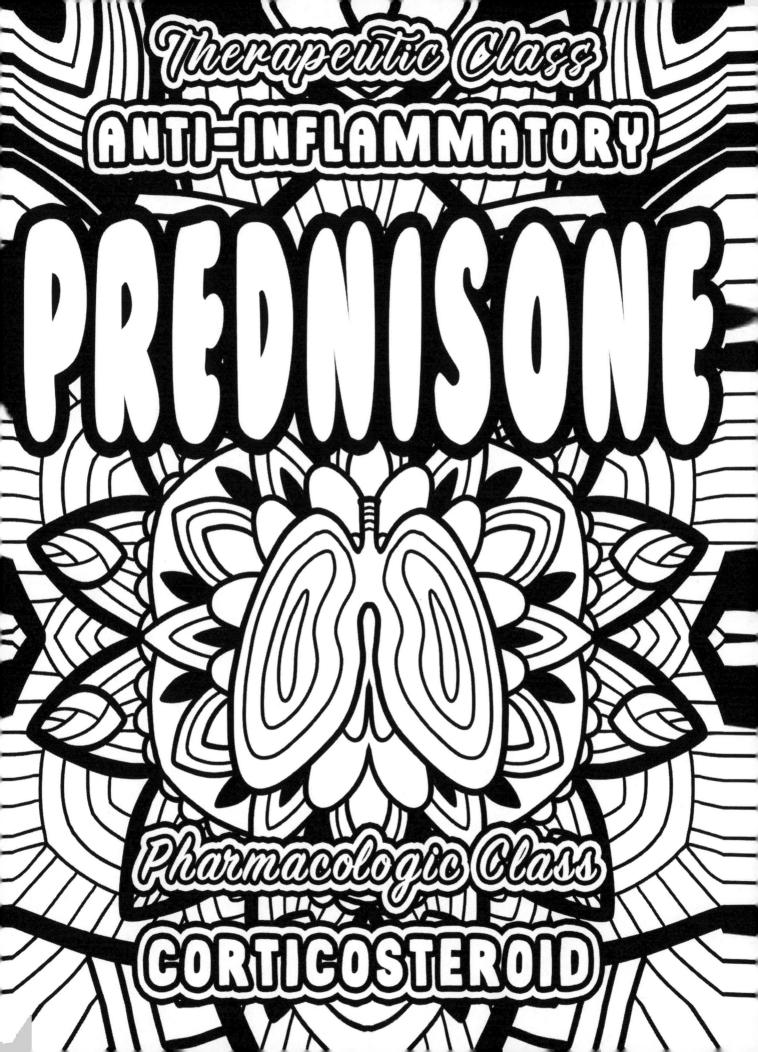

PREDNISONE

TRADE NAME
Omnipred

INDICATION
Asthma, COPD

NURSING CONSIDERATIONS
- Assess respiratory status
- Assess liver function
- Use caution with untreated infections and immunosuppressed patients
- DO NOT USE for acute asthma attacks

ACTION
Disrupts leukotriene activity, decreasing airway edema and smooth muscle constriction

NOTES

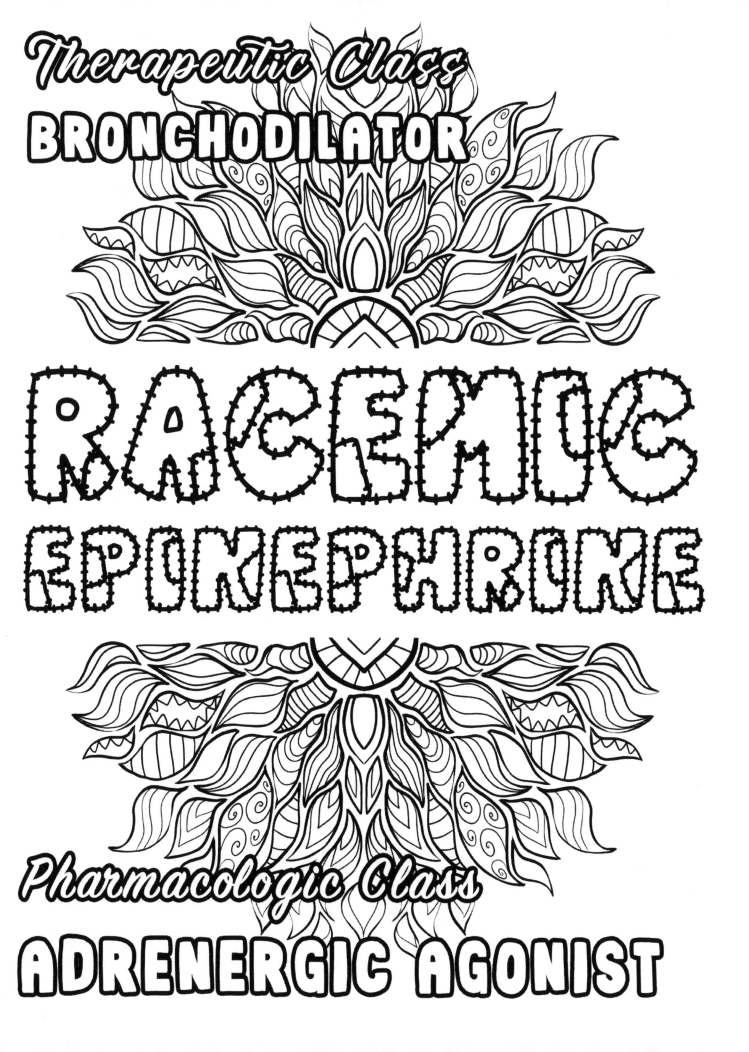

RACEMIC EPINEPHRINE

TRADE NAME
AsthmaNefrin

NURSING CONSIDERATIONS
- Monitor BP, pulse, and respirations
- Assess respiratory status
- Monitor for chest pain and palpitations
- Can decrease increase blood glucose levels

INDICATION
Acute Asthma, Croup

ACTION
Non-selective alpha and beta agonist, producing rapid bronchodilation

NOTES
_____
_____
_____
_____
_____
_____
_____
_____

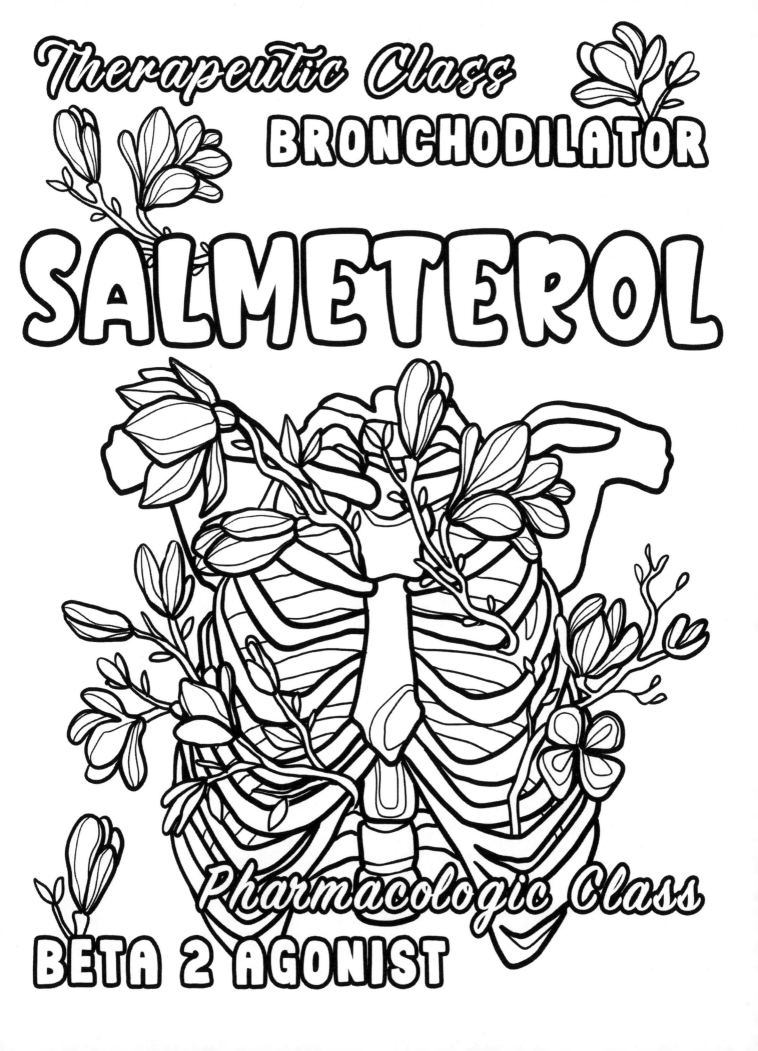

SALMETEROL

TRADE NAME
Serevent

INDICATION
Asthma, COPD, Exercise-Induced Bronchoconstriction

ACTION
Beta 2 adrenergic receptor agonist, leading to relaxation of the smooth muscles of the airway

NURSING CONSIDERATIONS
- Instruct patient to avoid overuse
- Can cause headache, palpitations, tachycardia, paradoxical bronchospasm
- Beta blockers may decrease effectiveness
- Assess respiratory status
- May increase blood glucose levels

NOTES
_____
_____
_____
_____
_____
_____
_____
_____
_____

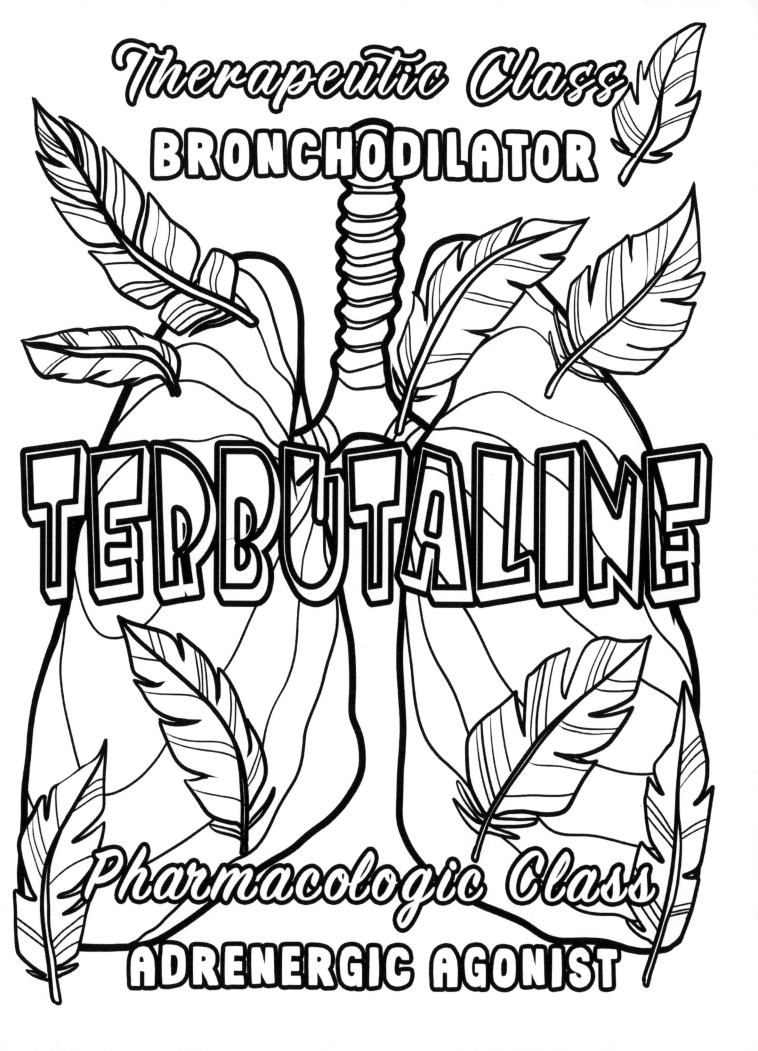

TERBUTALINE

TRADE NAME
Brethaire

INDICATION
Asthma, COPD, Pre-Term Labor

ACTION
Beta 2 adrenergic receptor agonist, leading to relaxation of the smooth muscles of the airway

NURSING CONSIDERATIONS
- May cause nervousness, restlessness, tremors
- Beta blockers may decrease effectiveness
- Assess respiratory status
- Monitor for hypoglycemia
- May cause hypokalemia
- Monitor maternal/fetal vital signs if using for pre-term labor

NOTES

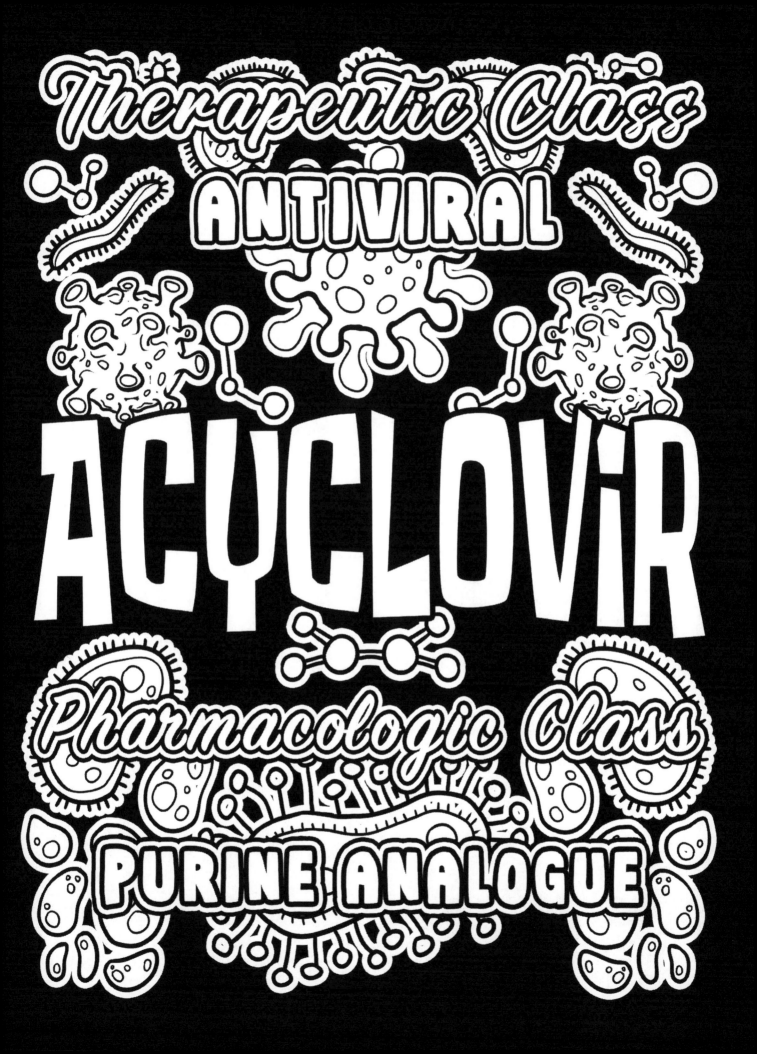

ACYCLOVIR

TRADE NAME
Zovirax

INDICATION
Genital Herpes, Herpes Zoster, Chicken Pox

ACTION
Bacteriostatic. Interferes with viral DNA synthesis.

NURSING CONSIDERATIONS
- May cause seizures, renal failure, Stevens-Johnson syndrome, thrombotic thrombocytopenic pupura syndrome, nausea/diarrhea, dizziness
- Monitor renal panel
- Assess lesions
- Instruct patient to use proper protection during sexual intercourse

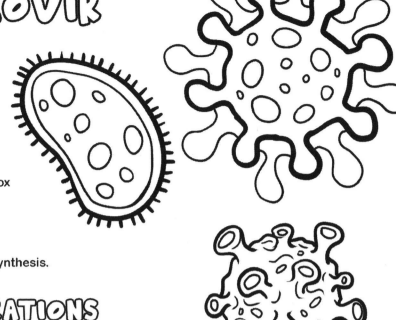

NOTES

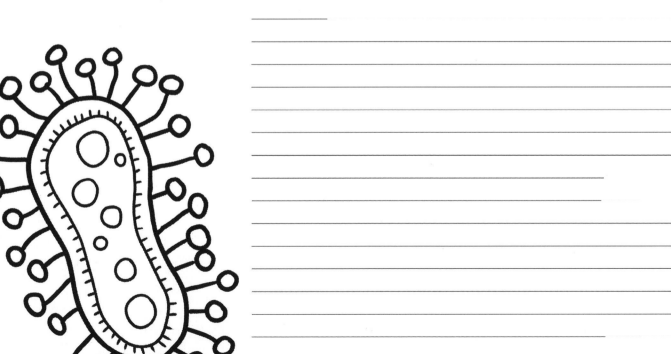

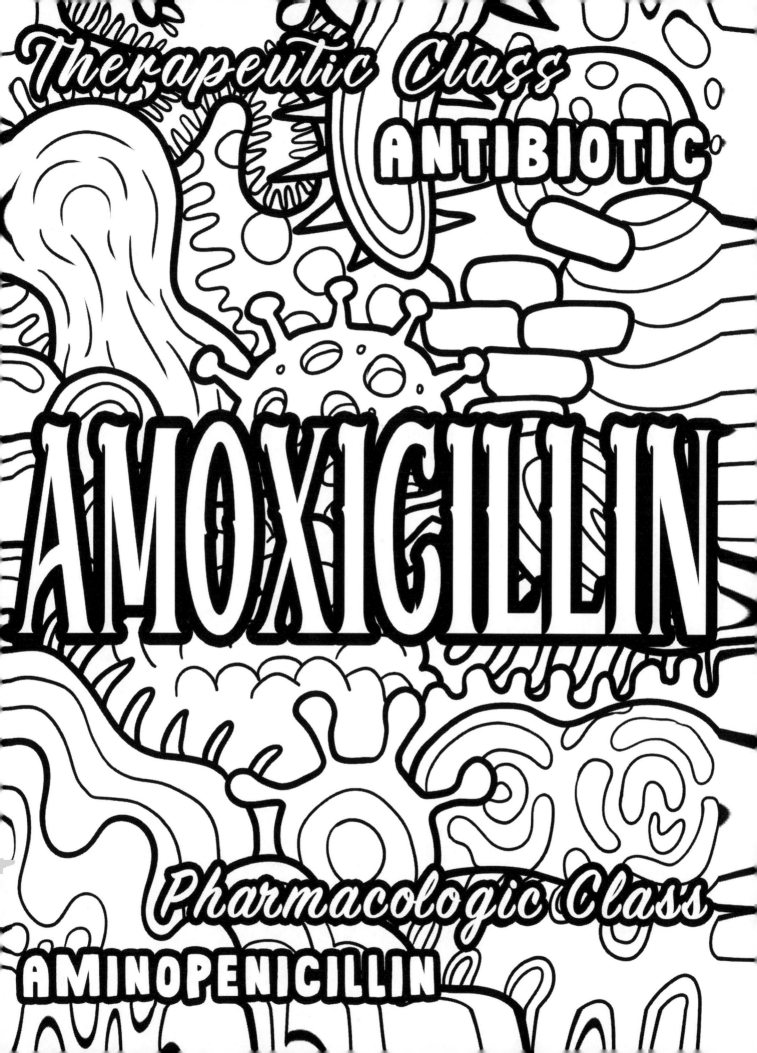

AMOXICILLIN

TRADE NAME

Moxatag

INDICATION

Skin Infections, Respiratory Infections, Sinusitis, Endocarditis, Lyme Disease

ACTION

Bactericidal. Inhibits synthesis of bacterial cell wall leading to cell death.

NURSING CONSIDERATIONS

- Contraindicated with penicillin allergy
- May cause seizures
- Assess for rash, anaphylaxis
- Excreted by kidneys – Monitor renal labs
- Monitor for diarrhea – Report bloody stool immediately

NOTES

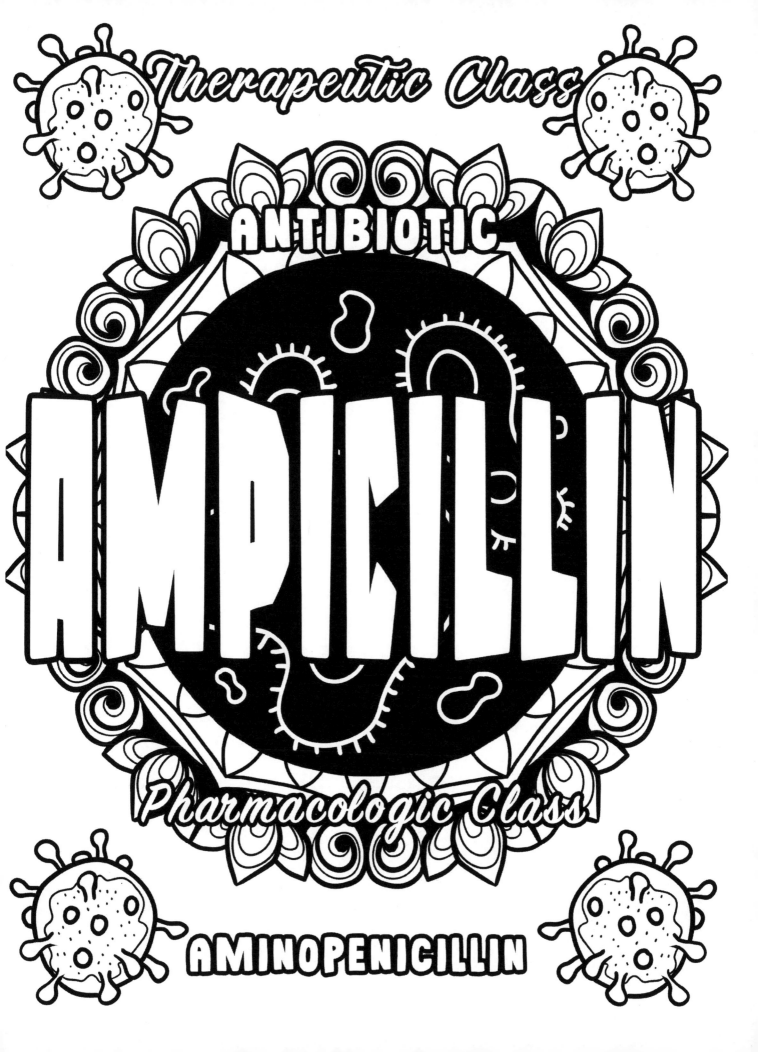

AMPICILLIN

TRADE NAME
Principen

INDICATION
Skin Infections, Respiratory Infections, Otitis Media, GU Infections, Meningitis, Septicemia

ACTION
Broader spectrum than penicillin. Bactericidal. Binds to bacterial cell wall leading to bacterial cell death.

NURSING CONSIDERATIONS
- Contraindicated with penicillin allergy
- May cause seizures, diarrhea, superinfection
- Monitor liver function tests
- Instruct patient on signs of superinfection: furry tongue, vaginal itching, loose and foul smelling stool
- DO NOT use with oral contraceptives

NOTES

Therapeutic Class

ANTIBIOTIC

AZITHROMYCIN

Pharmacologic Class

MACROLIDE

AZITHROMYCIN

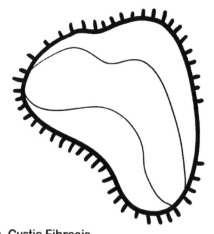

TRADE NAME
Zithromax

INDICATION
URI, Chronic Bronchitis, Otitis Media, Skin Infections, Various STI's, Endocarditis, Cystic Fibrosis

ACTION
Bactericidal. Inhibits bacterial protein synthesis leading to cell death.

NURSING CONSIDERATIONS
- May lead to pseudomembranous colitis, nausea/diarrhea, Stevens-Johnson syndrome, angioedema
- May increase risk of warfarin toxicity
- Instruct patient to notify physician for diarrhea, blood, or pus in stool
- Instruct patient to take medication exactly as prescribed

NOTES

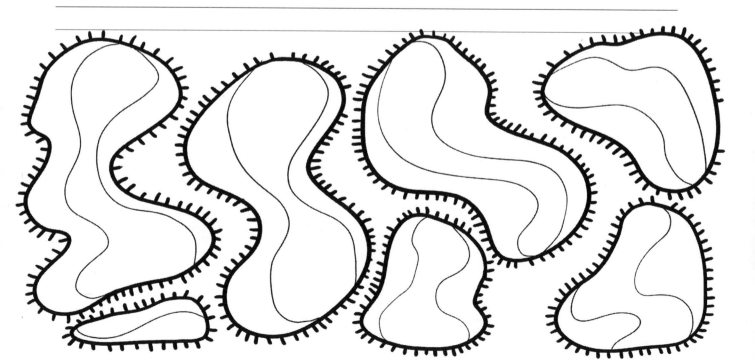

CEFACLOR

Therapeutic Class

ANTIBIOTIC

Pharmacologic Class

2ND GEN CEPHALOSPORIN

CEFACLOR

TRADE NAME
Ceclor

INDICATION
Respiratory Tract Infections, Skin Infections, Otitis Media

ACTION
Bactericidal. Binds to bacterial cell wall leading to cell death.

NURSING CONSIDERATIONS
- Contraindicated in cephalosporin allergy
- May lead to seizures, pseudomembranous colitis, diarrhea, phlebitis
- Obtain cultures prior to therapy
- Monitor bowel function
- May lead to superinfection

NOTES

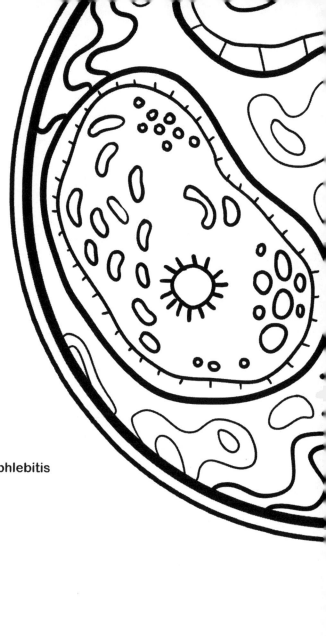
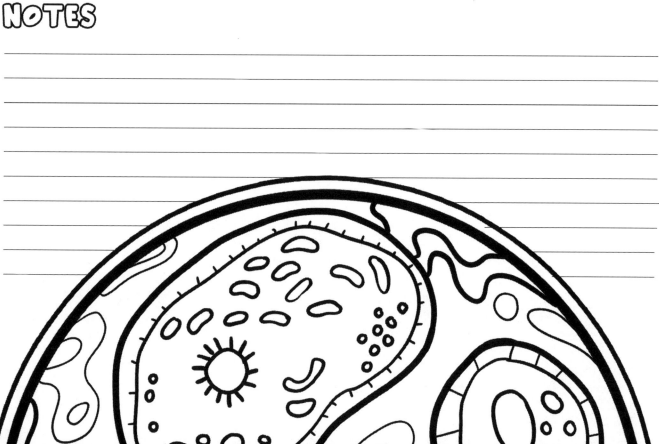

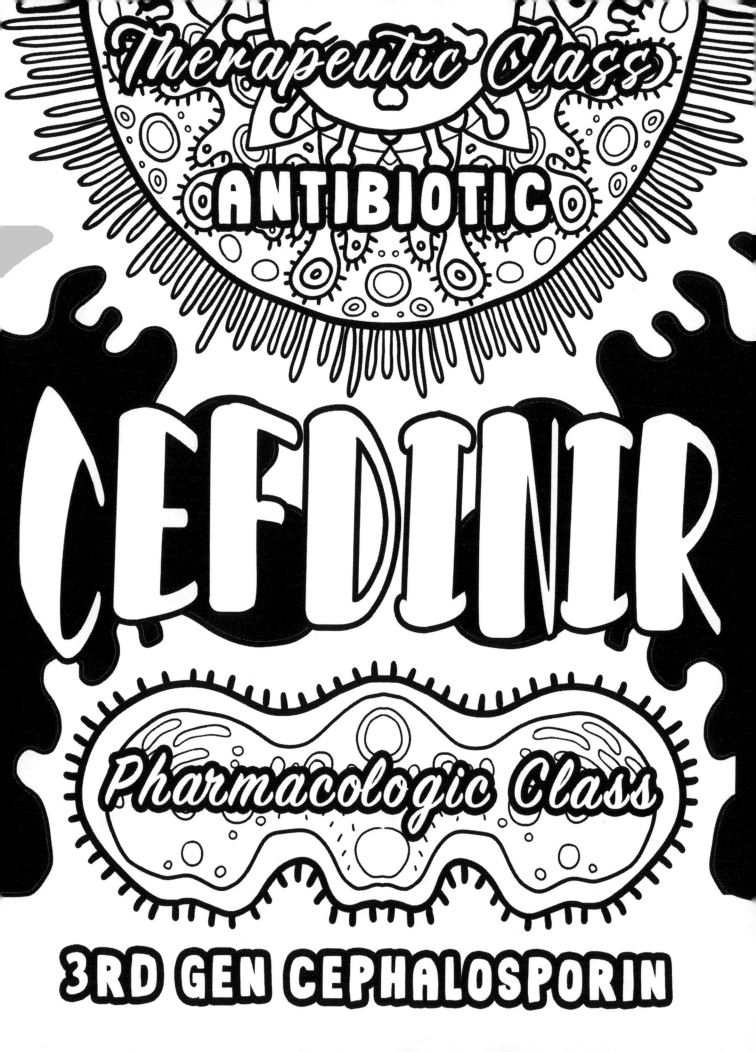

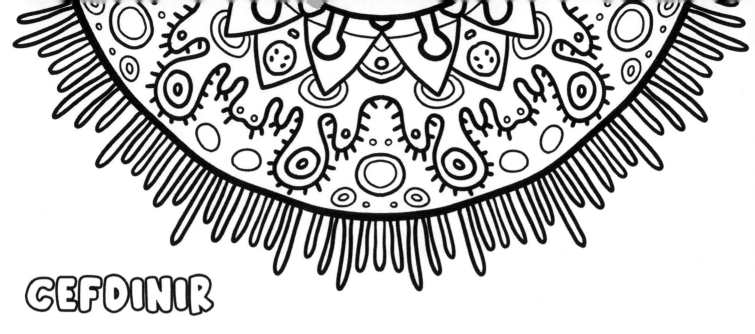

CEFDINIR

TRADE NAME
Omnicef

INDICATION
Skin Infections, Otitis Media

ACTION
Bactericidal. Binds to bacterial cell wall leading to cell death.

NURSING CONSIDERATIONS
- Contraindicated in cephalosporin allergy
- May lead to seizures, pseudomembranous colitis, diarrhea, phlebitis
- Obtain cultures prior to therapy
- Monitor bowel function, bleeding
- May lead to superinfection

NOTES

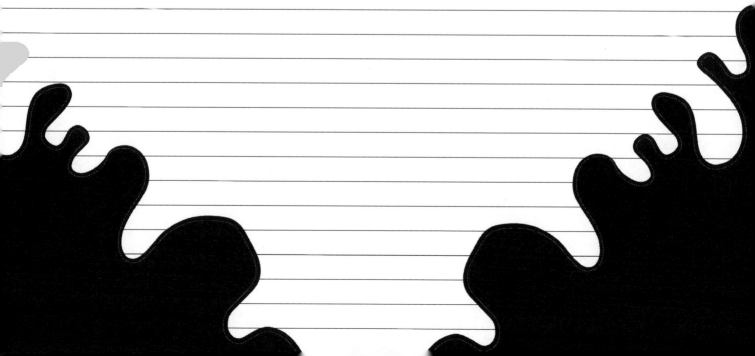

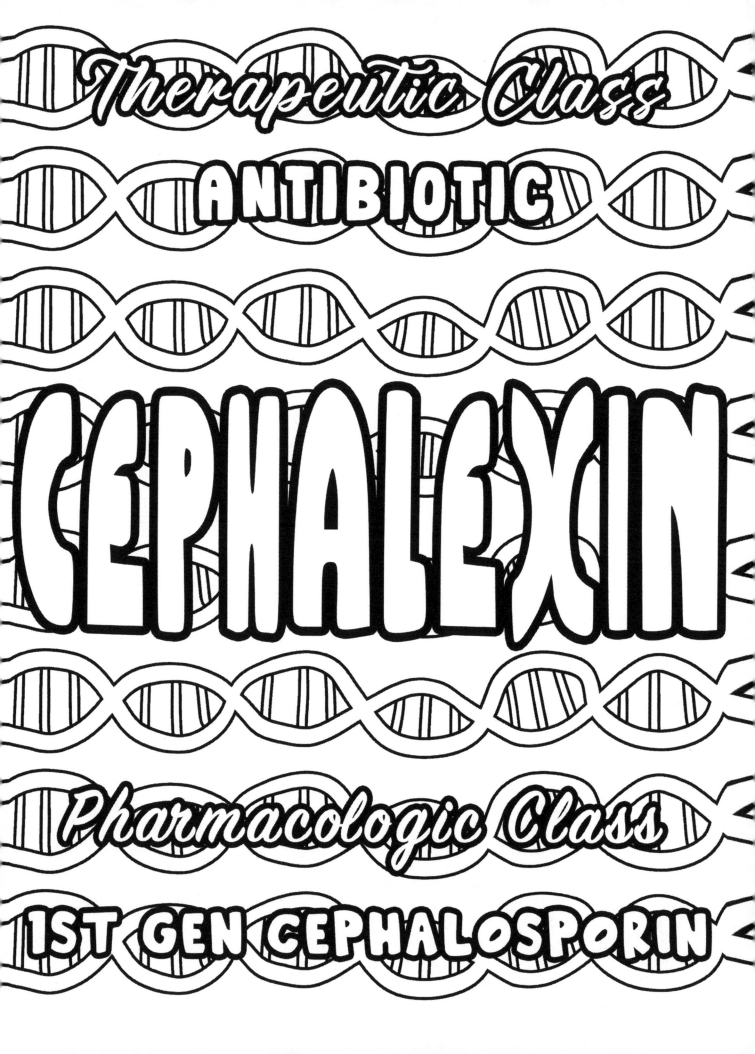

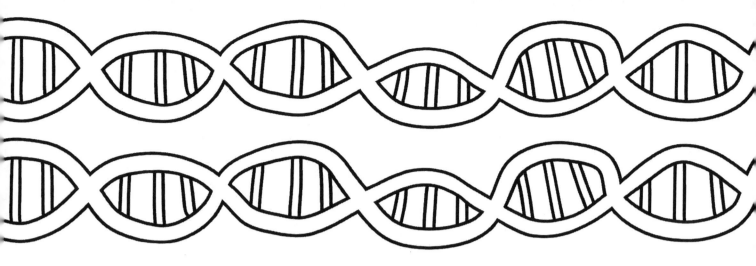

CEPHALEXIN

TRADE NAME
Keflex

INDICATION
Skin Infections, Pneumonia, UTI, Otitis Media

ACTION
Bactericidal. Binds to bacterial cell wall leading to cell death.

NURSING CONSIDERATIONS
- Contraindicated in cephalosporin allergy
- May lead to seizures, pseudomembranous colitis, diarrhea, phlebitis
- Obtain cultures prior to therapy
- Monitor bowel function
- May lead to superinfection, elevated liver enzymes

NOTES

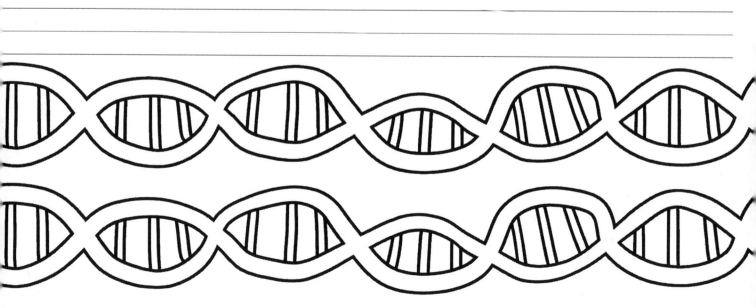

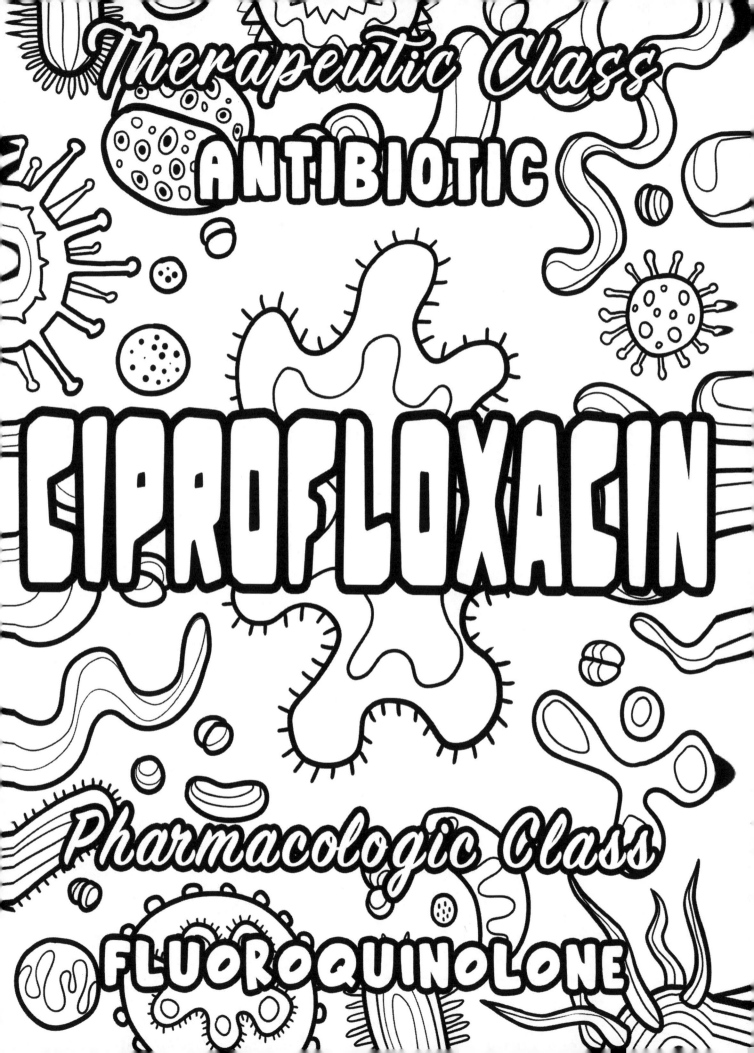

CIPROFLOXACIN

TRADE NAME
Cipro

INDICATION
Skin and Bone Infections, Pneumonia, UTI, Otitis Media, Gonorrhea, Abdominal Infections, Anthrax Exposure

ACTION
Bacteriostatic. Inhibits bacterial DNA synthesis.

NURSING CONSIDERATIONS
- May cause QT prolongation
- May lead to seizures, anaphylaxis, arrhythmias, pseudomembranous colitis, Stevens-Johnson syndrome
- May decrease effects of phenytoin
- Monitor renal panel, liver function tests

NOTES

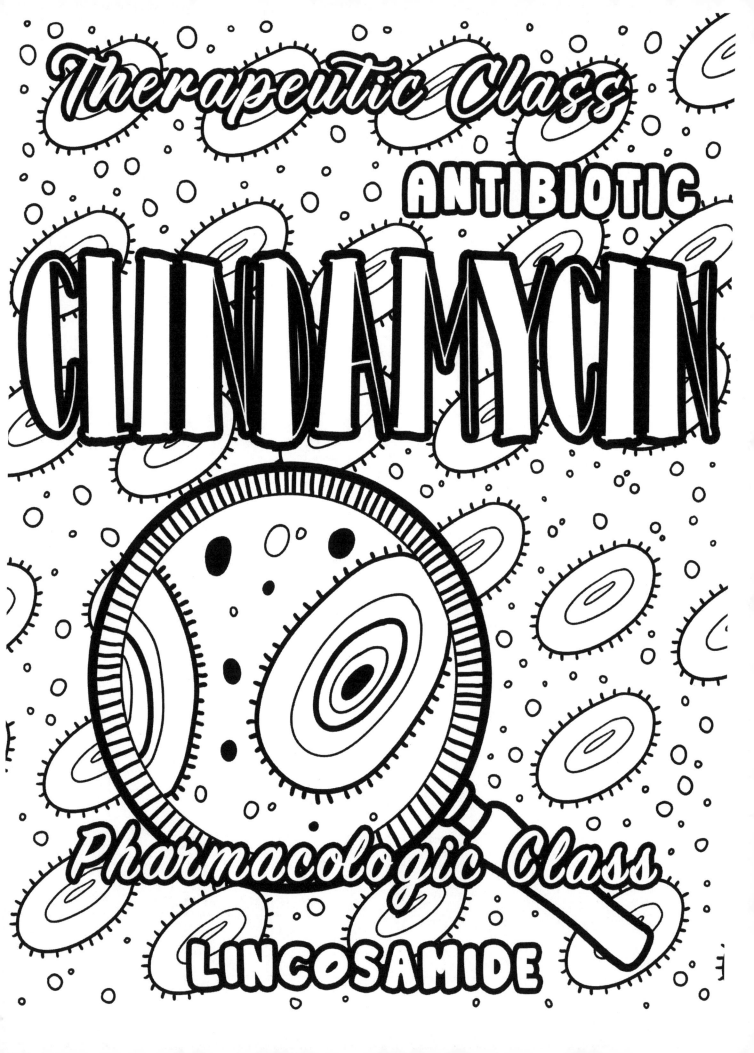

CLINDAMYCIN

TRADE NAME
Cleocin

INDICATION
Skin Infections, Respiratory Infections, Septicemia, Osteomyelitis, Abdominal Infections

ACTION
Bacteriostatic. Inhibits bacterial protein synthesis.

NURSING CONSIDERATIONS
- May lead to arrhythmias, pseudomembranous colitis, diarrhea, phlebitis
- Monitor bowel function
- Monitor liver function tests, CBC

NOTES

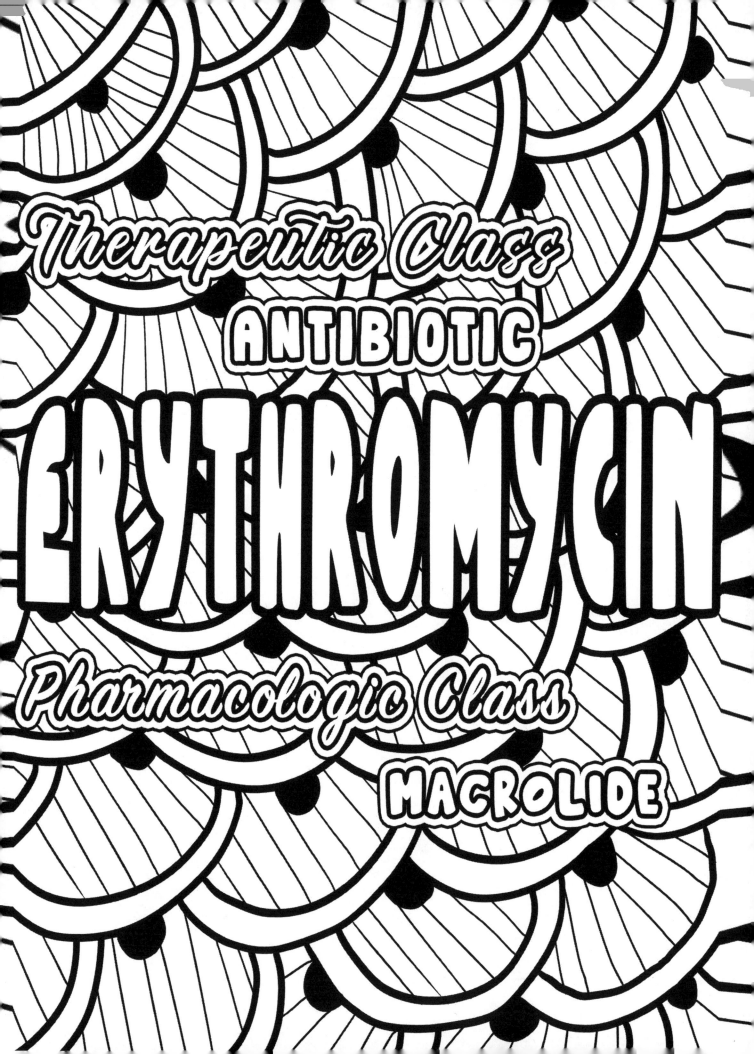

ERYTHROMYCIN

TRADE NAME

E-Mycin

INDICATION

Useful en lieu of penicillin when contraindicated. Respiratory Infections, Otitis Media, Skin Infections, Pertussis, Syphilis, Rheumatic Fever

ACTION

Bacteriostatic. Suppresses bacterial protein synthesis.

NURSING CONSIDERATIONS

- Causes QT prolongation, ventricular arrhythmias, diarrhea
- Monitor liver function tests
- Instruct patient not to share medication, complete prescription even if they feel better

NOTES

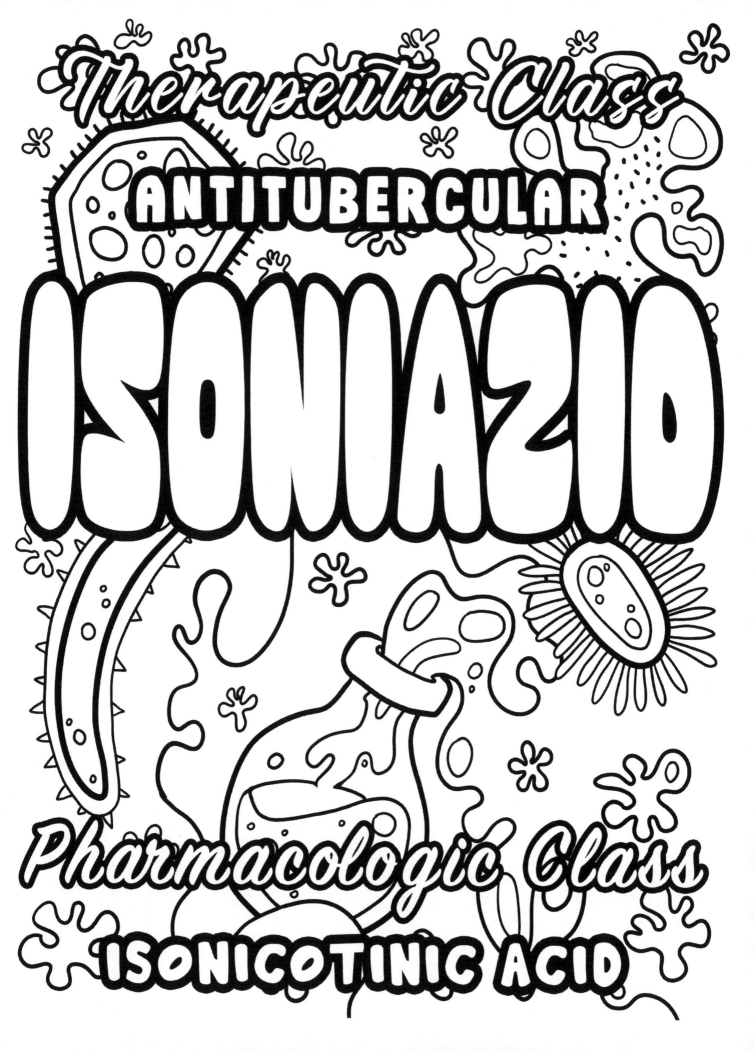

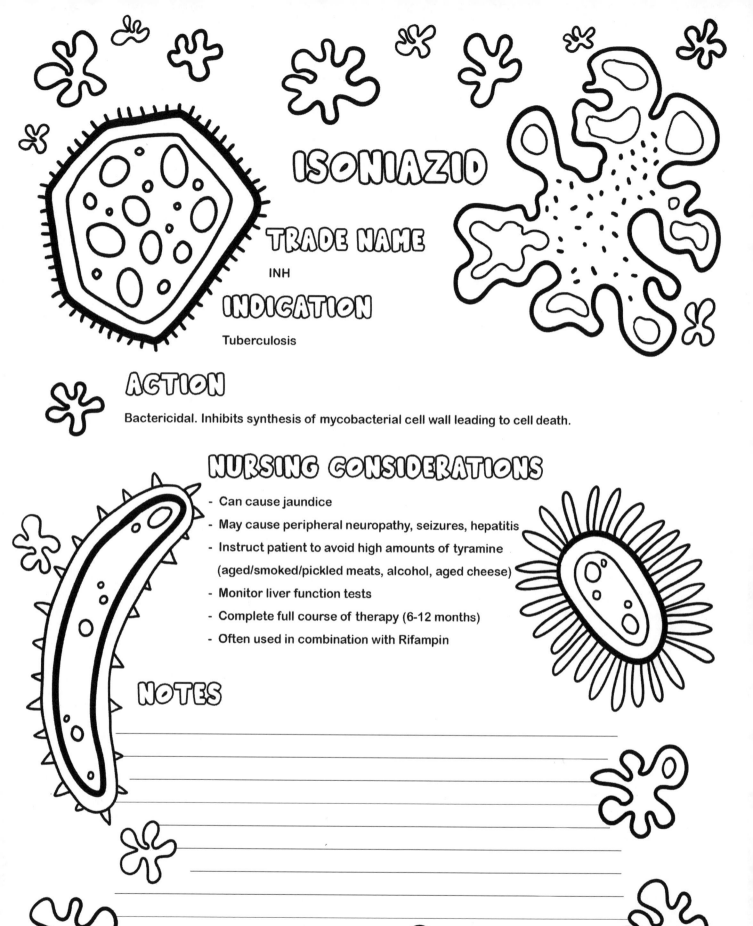

ISONIAZID

TRADE NAME
INH

INDICATION
Tuberculosis

ACTION
Bactericidal. Inhibits synthesis of mycobacterial cell wall leading to cell death.

NURSING CONSIDERATIONS
- Can cause jaundice
- May cause peripheral neuropathy, seizures, hepatitis
- Instruct patient to avoid high amounts of tyramine (aged/smoked/pickled meats, alcohol, aged cheese)
- Monitor liver function tests
- Complete full course of therapy (6-12 months)
- Often used in combination with Rifampin

NOTES

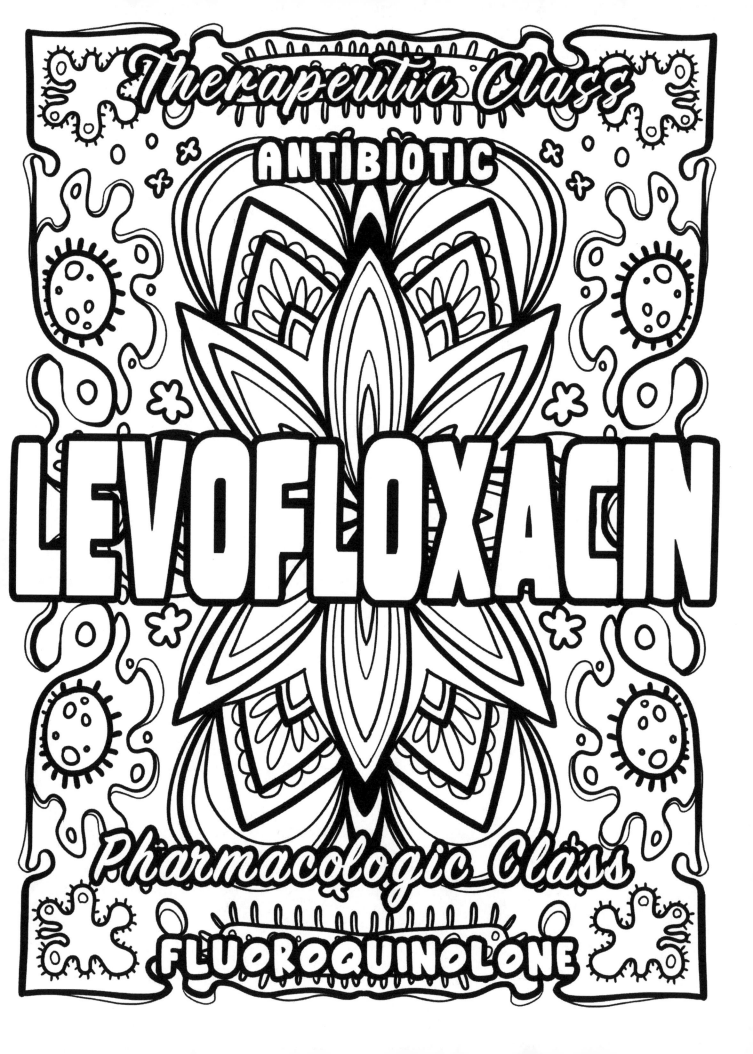

LEVOFLOXACIN

TRADE NAME
Levaquin

INDICATION
Urinary Tract Infection, Gonorrhea, Respiratory Tract Infections, Pneumonia, Skin and Bone Infections

ACTION
Bactericidal. Inhibits DNA synthesis in bacteria leading to cell death.

NURSING CONSIDERATIONS
- May cause QT prolongation, seizures, arrhythmias, pseudomembranous colitis, Stevens-Johnson syndrome
- May decrease effects of phenytoin
- Monitor liver function tests

NOTES

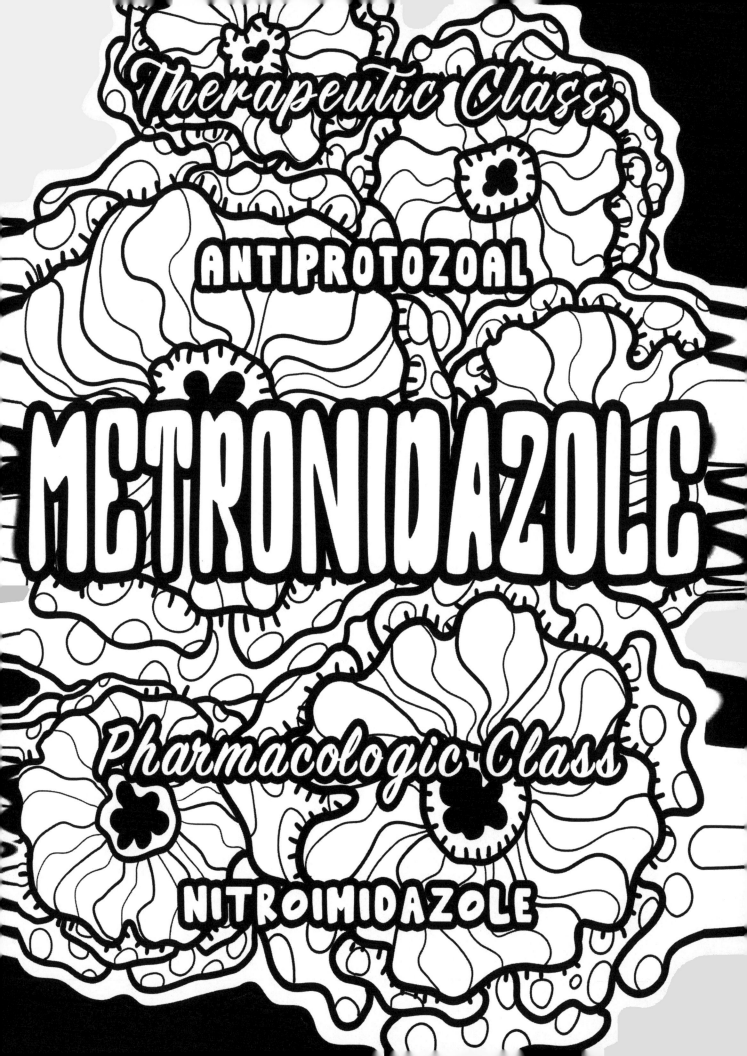

METRONIDAZOLE

TRADE NAME
Flagyl

INDICATION
Intra-Abdominal Infections, Gynecological Infections, Skin Infections, CNS Infections, Septicemia, Endocarditis, Amebic Liver Abcess, Peptic Ulcer Disease

ACTION
Bactericidal. Inhibits DNA and protein synthesis in bacteria leading to cell death.

NURSING CONSIDERATIONS
- DO NOT take with alcohol – May lead to disulfiram reaction
- Monitor neurological status: paresthesia, weakness, ataxia, seizures
- Monitor I's & O's, daily weights
- May alter liver enzyme tests

NOTES

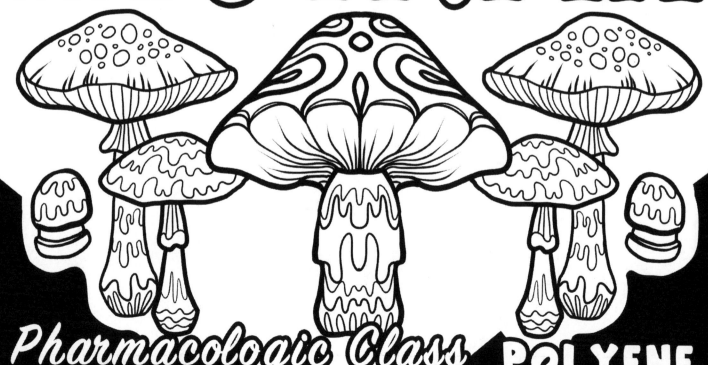

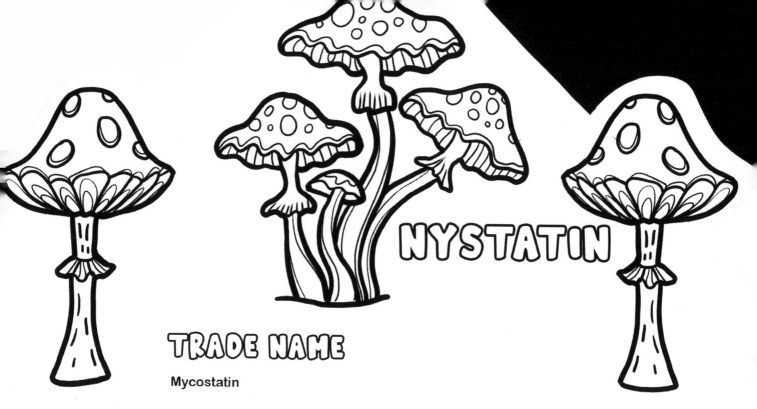

NYSTATIN

TRADE NAME
Mycostatin

INDICATION
Candidiasis, Denture Stomatitis

ACTION
Fungistatic and fungicidal. Causes leakage of fungal cell contents.

NURSING CONSIDERATIONS
- May cause diarrhea, nausea/vomiting
- Can be used to soak dentures
- Assess mucus membranes

NOTES

Therapeutic Class
ANTITUBERCULAR

RIFAMPIN

Pharmacologic Class
RIFAMYCIN

RIFAMPIN

TRADE NAME
Rimactane

INDICATION
Tuberculosis

ACTION
Bactericidal. Inhibits bacterial RNA synthesis.

NURSING CONSIDERATIONS
- Can turn body fluids red
- May cause diarrhea, nausea/vomiting, confusion
- Assess lung sounds and sputum characteristics
- Evaluate renal and liver function tests
- Instruct patient not to skip or double dose
- Complete full course of therapy (6-12 months)

NOTES

Therapeutic Class

ANTIBIOTIC

TETRACYCLINE

Pharmacologic Class

TETRACYCLINE

TETRACYCLINE

TRADE NAME
Doxycycline

INDICATION
Useful en lieu of penicillin for Gonorrhea, Syphilis, Chronic Bronchitis

ACTION
Bacteriostatic. Inhibits bacterial protein synthesis.

NURSING CONSIDERATIONS
- Use caution in setting of liver impairment
- May cause pseudomembranous colitis, diarrhea, nausea/vomiting, photosensitivity, rash
- May increase effects of warfarin
- Evaluate renal and liver function tests
- Instruct patient to complete entire course

NOTES

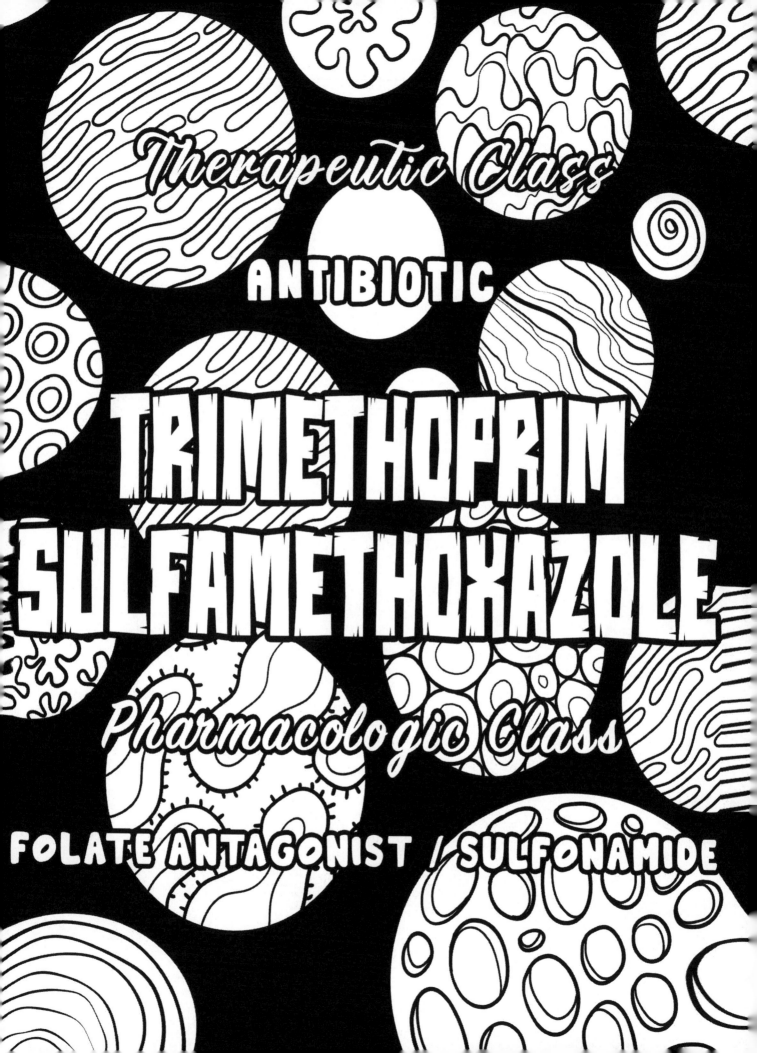

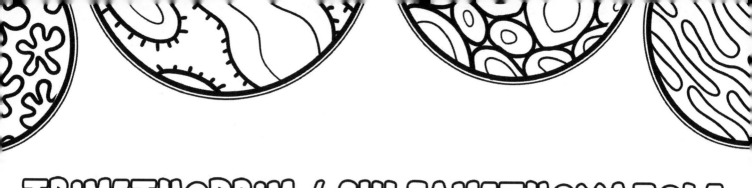

TRIMETHOPRIM / SULFAMETHOXAZOLE

TRADE NAME
Bactrim / TMP-SMZ

INDICATION
Bronchitis, UTI, Diarrhea, Pneumonia

ACTION
Bactericidal. Prevents bacterial metabolism of folic acid.

NURSING CONSIDERATIONS
- May cause renal damages, Steven-Johnson syndrome
- May cause pseudomembranous colitis, diarrhea, nausea/vomiting, rash
- Contraindicated with sulfa allergies
- Monitor I's & O's
- Instruct patient to drink 8-10 glasses of water a day

NOTES

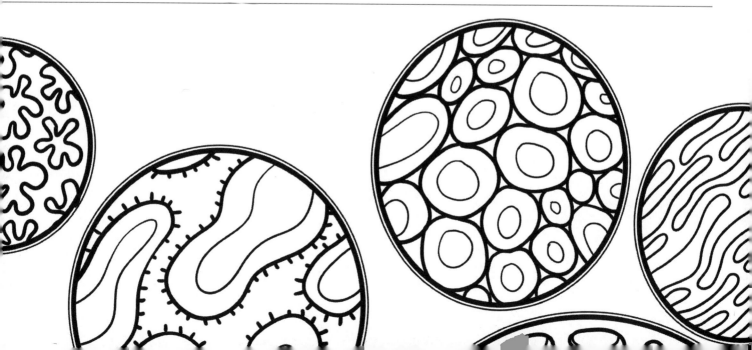

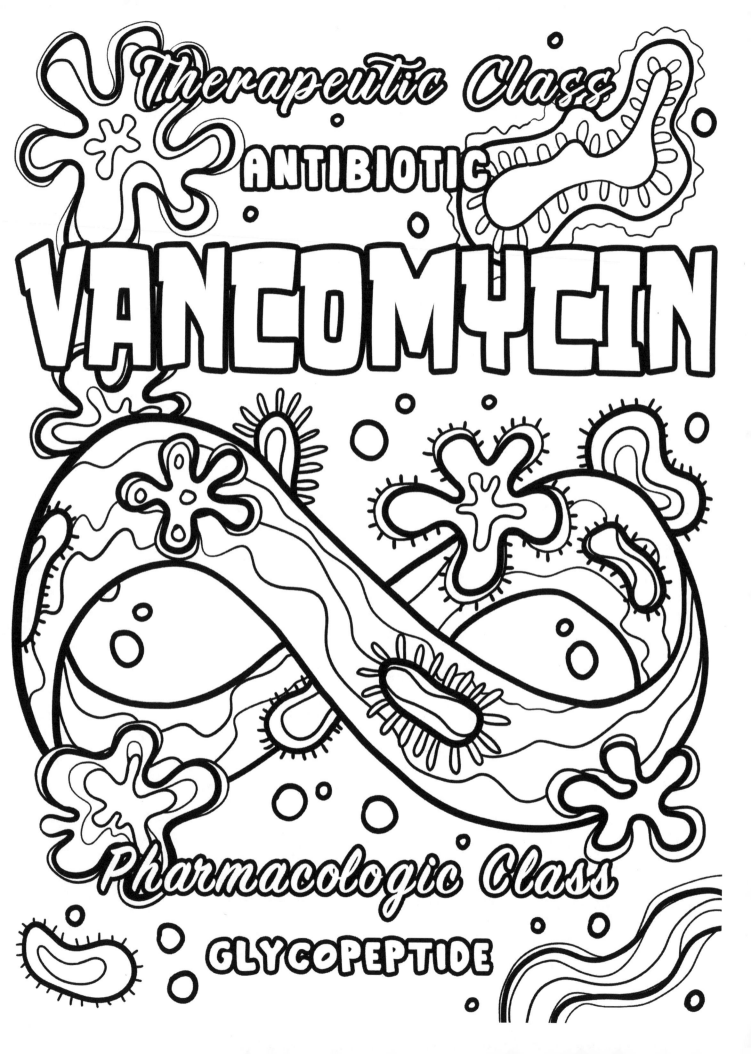

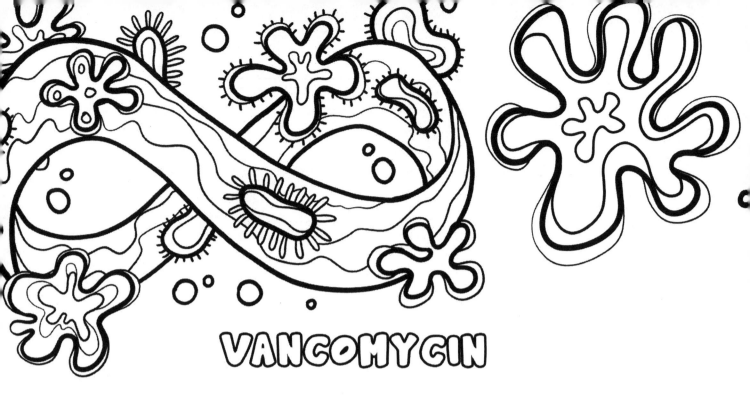

VANCOMYCIN

TRADE NAME
Vancocin

INDICATION
Life Threatening Infections, Sepsis

ACTION
Bactericidal. Prevents bacterial cell wall synthesis.

NURSING CONSIDERATIONS
- Can cause ototoxicity, nausea/vomiting, nephrotoxicity, anaphylaxis, red-man syndrome
- Monitor blood pressure
- DOSE DEPENDENT: Draw serum trough levels frequently
- Administer over at least 60 minutes to avoid skin irritation

NOTES

_____
_____
_____
_____
_____
_____
_____
_____
_____

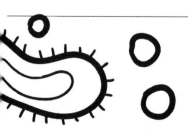
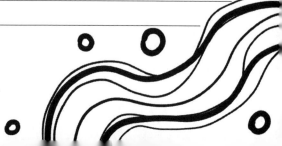

COLOR TEST PAGE

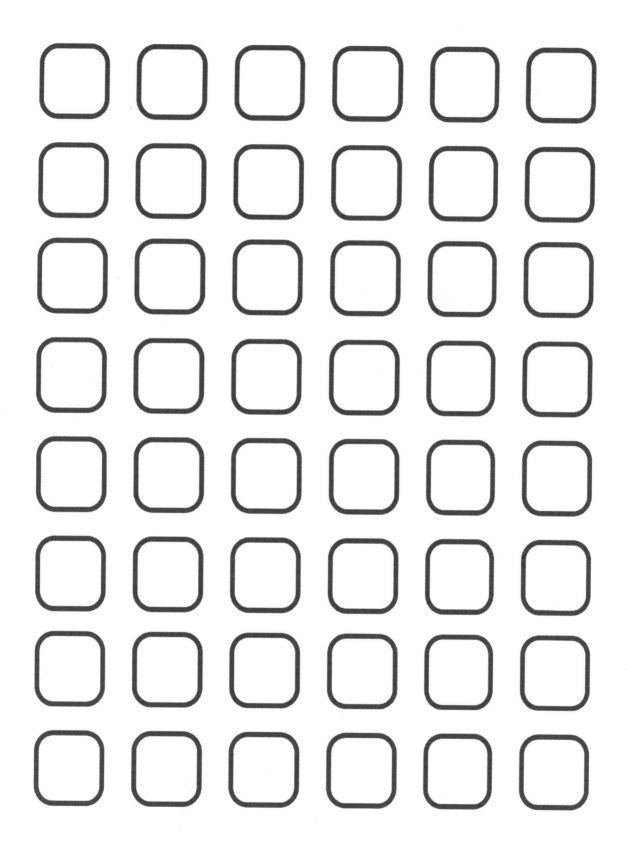

Made in the USA
Columbia, SC
10 December 2024